Sensory Processing Disorder

Practical Parenting Techniques for Developing Self-Assurance, Adaptability, Relationships, and Success with SPD Kids

Michele L. Valdez.

Introducing the exclusive and captivating world of Michele L. Valdez. Immerse yourself in the timeless elegance and creativity that defines our brand. Experience the unparalleled craftsmanship and attention to detail that sets us apart. Discover the essence of sophistication and style with our exquisite collection.

Table of Contents

Preface

Are you a teacher, caregiver, or parent who wants to provide kids with sensory processing disorder (SPD) the tools they need to succeed? There's nowhere else to look! A novel method to controlling SPD is provided by Sensory Solutions: Unlocking Your Child's Potential, which combines the most recent research with useful tactics catered to specific requirements. This book provides a ray of hope and empowerment for families overcoming the difficulties caused by sensory processing differences—it's not just another on SPD.

Revealing the Adventure

Envision an environment where the distinct sensory requirements of your child are not perceived as hindrances, but rather as chances for advancement and maturation. We set out on a voyage of exploration at Sensory Solutions, releasing each child's full potential. This book provides a path to confidently and compassionately manage the intricacies of sensory processing difficulties by taking a comprehensive approach that takes into account the social, emotional, and physical components of SPD.

Empowerment via Comprehension

The power of knowledge is one of Sensory Solutions' pillars. Understanding, in our opinion, is the first step toward empowerment. For this reason, we explore the science underlying sensory processing, demystifying difficult ideas and providing useful advice that will enable you to speak out for your child's special needs. We offer concise explanations and practical advice on everything from sensory discrimination to sensory modulation, enabling you to be your child's strongest supporter as they pursue success.

Tailor-Made Success Strategies

Since each child with SPD is different, there is no one-size-fits-all method for managing their sensory intake. Understanding that every child is unique, Sensory Solutions provides individualized techniques based on each child's unique sensory profile. Whether your child is sensitive to sensory input, avoids it, or is seeking it out, we offer helpful advice and strategies to help them succeed in daily life. You'll find a multitude of options to assist your child's sensory journey, ranging from ambient adjustments to sensory diets.

Developing Adaptability and Adaptability

Sensory Solutions strives to help children with SPD develop resilience beyond just survival. Every obstacle is a chance for development, and we provide them the tools they need to bravely and confidently accept who they are. We demonstrate the transforming power of resilience in conquering challenges and succeeding via true stories and motivational anecdotes. We provide kids with the resources they need to face life's obstacles head-on, whether they are in the classroom or on the playground: resilience and grace.

Creating a Supporting Community

The goal of creating a supportive network for families with children with SPD is the foundation of Sensory Solutions. We cordially encourage you to embark with us on this life-changing trip, acknowledging that no journey is meant to be taken alone. We offer a platform for families to connect, share resources, and find comfort in the knowing that they are not alone through online forums, support groups, and networking events. By working together, we can make a world in which all children with SPD are accepted, understood, and valued for their unique identities.

Make the Initial Move in the Direction of Change

Are you prepared to start your child on a path of resilience and empowerment and to help them reach their full potential? Order your copy of Sensory Solutions: Unlocking Your Child's Potential today to take the first step. This book is your roadmap to successfully and compassionately managing the difficulties of SPD, whether you're a parent, caregiver, or educator. Come along with us as we turn obstacles into chances and enable kids with sensory processing disorders to flourish in a society that values their individual talents and capabilities. One sensory solution at a time, we can all work together to change things.

Introduction

Explore the complex realm of sensory processing difficulties on a transforming journey with "Sensory Processing Disorder: Navigating Life's Spectrum." With empathy and knowledge, Michele L. Valdez provides a road map for appreciating and comprehending the wide range of sensory experiences.

This book is a ray of empowerment and optimism for people navigating their own sensory landscapes or stressed parents looking for comfort. Dive into doable tactics designed to help each person reach their full potential while promoting self-awareness and resilience.

Learn about comprehensive strategies that go beyond conventional limits and close the gap between sensory variations and the wider range of neurodiversity. Through perceptive stories and research-backed advice, Michele L. Valdez shows the route toward inclusivity and acceptance.

This book is a lifeline for anyone dealing with sensory issues, whether they are educators, caregivers, or individuals themselves. It provides encouragement, affirmation, and practical solutions. With the help of "Sensory Processing Disorder: Navigating Life's Spectrum," embrace the path of comprehending and appreciating sensory diversity.

Sensory Processing Disorder, also known as SPD, can present unique challenges for individuals. It is important to recognize and support neurodiversity, as well as provide caregiver support. Taking a holistic approach that emphasizes acceptance, inclusion, and resilience can empower individuals with SPD. Exploring sensory experiences and implementing practical strategies can help foster understanding and promote diversity. Self-discovery and compassion are key in navigating the world with SPD.

Chapter 1

Symptoms of Sensory Processing Disorder

Sensory Processing Disorder may affect one sense, like hearing, touch, or taste. Or it might influence multiple senses. And folks could be over or under-responsive to the items they end up having. Like many illnesses, the symptoms of sensory control disorder exist around the spectrum.

In a few children, for instance, the sound from the leaf blower away from window might lead these to vomit or dive beneath the table. They could scream when handled. They could recoil from your textures of particular foodstuffs. But others appear unresponsive to anything around them. They could neglect to respond to extreme warmth or chills and even pain.

Many children with sensory processing disorder begin as fussy babies who become stressed because they grow older. These kids often don't deal well with change. They could frequently toss tantrums or have meltdowns. Many children have symptoms like these occasionally. But therapists take a look at an analysis of Sensory Digesting Disorder when the symptoms become severe enough with an influence on normal working and disrupt living.

Causes of Sensory Processing Disorder

The exact reason behind sensory processing problems isn't identified. But a study of some selected twins showed that hypersensitivity to light and sound may have a considerable genetic component.

Other experiments display that children with sensory processing disorders have irregular brain activity if they are simultaneously put through light and sound.

Still, additional experiments show that children with sensory processing problems will continue to respond highly to a stroke within the hand or a loud sound, while other children quickly become accustomed to the sensations.

Treatment for Sensory Processing Disorder

Many families with an affected child find it hard to get help. That's because sensory processing disorder isn't an acknowledged medical diagnosis at this time.

Regardless of the insufficient widely accepted diagnostic requirements, occupational therapists commonly discover and treat children and adults with sensory digesting problems.

However, generally, it entails assisting children do better at activities they're generally bad at and helping them become accustomed to things they cannot tolerate.

Treatment for sensory processing problems is known as Sensory Integration. The goal of sensory integration is usually to engage a youngster in an excellent, playful way so they could work out how to respond appropriately and function more normally.

One sort of therapy is known as the Developmental, Person Difference, Relationship-based (DIR) model. The procedure originated through Stanley Greenspan, MD, and Serena Wieder, Ph.D. A substantial area of the therapy may be the "floor-time" technique. The technique involves multiple classes of play with a child and father or mother. The fun periods last about 20 minutes.

Through the sessions, parents are first asked to look at the child's lead, even if the playtime behavior isn't typical. These activities permit the father or mother to "enter" the child's world.

That is accompanied by another phase, where parents utilize the play sessions to create challenges for a child. The issues support pull a child into what Greenspan calls a "distributed" world using the father or mother. And the down sides produce opportunities for a child to comprehend essential skills in areas such as for example:

- Relating.

- Communicating.

- Thinking.

The classes are tailored towards the child's needs. For instance, if a child would under-react to touch and audio, the parent should be very dynamic through the next stage from the fun classes. If a child overreacts to touch and sound, the parent ought to be more calming.

Indicators of Sensory Processing Disorder

Ask parents of kids with learning and behavioral disorders if their children experience problems with sensory disorder, and most of these will answer having a resounding "yes." Though it is broadly accepted that the majority of children with Autism Spectrum Disorders have trouble processing sensory insight, the actual fact that children who aren't for the spectrum also experience these issues to differing degrees happens to be analyzed more carefully from the special need community. While all children can appear quirky or particular about their needs and wants, children with Sensory Processing Disorder (also called Sensory Integration Dysfunction) may also be severely experiencing their sensory choices it inhibits their everyday activities. Sensory issues are often regarded as either hypersensitivity (over-responsiveness) or hyposensitivity (under-responsiveness) to sensory stimuli. Here are some common indicators of Sensory Processing Disorder.

Hypersensitivities to sensory insight range from:

- Extreme response to or nervous about sudden, high-pitched, noisy, or metallic noises like flushing toilets, clanking silverware, or other sounds that appear inoffensive to others.

- May see or end up being distracted by background sounds that others don't actually hear.

- Fearful of surprise touch, avoids hugs and cuddling despite having familiar adults.

- Seems fearful of crowds or avoids taking a stand near others.

- Doesn't just like a game of label and it is overly fearful of swings and playground equipment.

- Extremely fearful of climbing or falling, despite the fact that there is no actual danger, i.e., doesn't like his or her feet to become off underneath.

- Offers poor balance, may fall often.

- Hypo-sensitivities to sensory insight range from:

- A continuous need to touch people or textures, despite the fact that it's inappropriate to do this.

- Doesn't realise personal space despite the fact that same-age peers are old enough to grasp it.

- Clumsy and uncoordinated movements.

- Exceptionally high tolerance for or indifference to pain.

- Often harms other children and pets when playing, i.e., doesn't realise his strengths and weaknesses.

- Is usually quite fidgety and struggling to sit still, enjoys movement-based play like content spinning, jumping, etc.

- Is apparently a "thrill seeker" and may end up being dangerous sometimes.

Chapter 2

A Comprehensive Overview of Sensory Processing Disorders

The inability to properly organize and respond to data gathered from the senses is known as sensory processing difficulties. Children afflicted with these conditions may have an excess of or deficit in sensory insight, or even both.

In what ways can sensory processing dysfunction manifest itself?

Problems with sensory data regulation are what this name describes. These conditions, which are sometimes known as Sensory Integration Disorder or Sensory Digestive Disorder, can have a major impact on daily functioning and learning.

Attention Deficit/Hyperactivity Disorder Fact Sheet

- Get a fact sheet on sensory digestion problems; it's only one page long.

This summary can address some of the more fundamental questions you may have regarding these intricate matters. You'll find professional opinions and guidance, practical applications at home, and details on the finest educational strategies for your child.

You should educate yourself on what to do and where to receive assistance if you suspect your child has sensory control issues. And if you've just learned that your child has these issues, figure out what to do next.

So, what exactly is a Spectrum Disorder?

It can be difficult for certain people's brains to process and make sense of sensory data. Some environments, sounds, scents, and textures can cause what is known as "sensory overload." Many things can make children feel anxious and irritated, including bright lights, sudden noises, particular textures in food, and itchy clothes.

There are two main categories of sensory processing issues, and many children suffer from both. The most important one is hypersensitivity, or being overly sensitive. As a result, some children may develop a phobia of sensory input, which causes them to avoid it. Hyposensitivity, or under-sensitivity, is the other. As a result, children develop a need for more sensory stimulation and start seeking it out.

- A Fact Sheet on Dyslexia

Find out what a mother discovered about her child's sensory difficulties.

Children that struggle with sensory processing are often overly sensitive. Those emotions that they find unbearable are avoided.

But rather than less, many children want more sensory stimulation. They may express a desire to physically engage with objects, people, and pressure. They may have an abnormally high tolerance for pain and be undersensitive to it. So kids can opt to play rough instead of recognizing when they're hurting someone.

A child may exhibit symptoms of both sensory avoidance and desire in the same child. Some of their emotions may be exaggerated, while others may go unnoticed. In addition, a child's reactions to the same environment or set of circumstances can vary throughout the day and even from one day to the next.

There is no one learning disability that includes sensory processing difficulties. But they may still make a big splash when it comes to education.

Early Warning Signs of Sensory Processing Disorder

Whether you or your child's educator notice anything depends on two factors. Your child's sensory awareness is the initial and foremost trigger. The kind of your child's sensory digestion difficulty is a potential second factor.

Sensory Deprivation

Many things can trigger an allergic reaction in children who are sensory avoidant. Some examples include things like certain foods' scents or textures, uncomfortable clothing, overcrowding, and loud noises. Reactions can often be rather strong, regardless of the consequence.

Sensory meltdowns can occur when there is an excess of

senses. Because they are under the child's control, they differ greatly from tantrums.

Additional indicators that your child may exhibit are:

- Seeks for quiet areas in busy, chaotic environments.

- Startled quickly by loud noises.

- Overwhelmed by intense light.

- Won't put on shoes that itch or cause any other kind of discomfort.

- Refrains from hugging or squeezing individuals.

- Extreme sensitivity to certain foods due to their texture or aroma.

- Eats only freshly prepared items and has a limited diet of chosen foods.

Reacts negatively to even minor changes in program or environment and shies away from trying anything new.

The first five senses—sight, smell, taste, touch, and sound—are not the only ones that contribute to sensory data. The less well-known sense of interoception allows you to become aware of and engage with your internal experiences. Toilet training or having a healthy pain threshold could be more challenging for children with impaired interoception.

Children who have problems with one or more of their senses may also have trouble with the other or with spatial orientation (the vestibular sense) or with bodily awareness (proprioception). When children avoid certain stimuli, it can be difficult to gauge how they interact with others and their surroundings. Another option is that they are careful when utilizing playground equipment, such as the swings.

Exploring the Senses

The inverse is true for children who lack sensory understanding. They usually necessitate motion. On top of that, they might probe for indications of preferences for things like sourness or heat, as well as tactile touch and pressure.

Additional symptoms that may manifest in your child at

various ages include the following:

- Repeatedly handles roughhousing and demands physical risks

- Continually touches objects

- More pain tolerance

- Frequently wriggles and fidgets

- Always on the go

- Invades the personal space of many persons

- Easily distracted or anxious

- Definitely awkward and uncoordinated

The manner a youngster is coping or self-regulating at any given moment determines whether they are "sensory seeking" in certain situations and "sensory staying away" in others. Because of this, learning your child's reactions and being prepared for potential triggers is of the utmost importance.

A Few Other Possible Co-Occurring Disorders with

Sensory Processing Disorders

On their own, sensory processing abnormalities cannot be diagnosed. But ADHD and Autism are common co-occurring disorders. Children with sensory processing disorders are not necessarily autistic or ADHD. Finally, I had established the concept of sensory overload and had a breakdown.

Severe difficulties with sensory regulation could mimic many of the signs of attention deficit hyperactivity disorder. Example: children with one of the conditions may need to be on the go all the time. But the reasons would differ.

Issues with sensory processing in children may mimic those in attention deficit hyperactivity disorder (ADHD). We must discover the reasons why children with sensory impairments may experience stress.

Some Hypothesized Reasons for Sensory Processing Disorders

Scientists are interested in the biologically based causes

of these problems. These disorders may run in families, according to some studies. Delivery issues and other environmental considerations will also be examined by experts. However, sensory digestion problems have no identified cause as of yet.

The presence of sensory impairments is common in both autism and ADHD. But they aren't the ones that cause them.

Methods for Diagnosing Sensory Processing Disorders

Although they are commonly referred to as "sensory processing disorder," sensory processing dysfunctions are not a recognized medical diagnosis. "Your kid provides trouble processing sensory information," is one such statement you could hear from a professional examiner.

Three Easy Recipes for Sensory-Friendly Slime

In order to diagnose sensory processing disorders, medical experts might administer a battery of tests. Among these, you can find the Sensory Control Measure (SPM) checklist and the Sensory Integration and Praxis

Assessments (SIPA).

However, in most cases, the actions that children exhibit are obvious and noticeable. Seeing your child and making notes to discuss with professionals who can diagnose their problems is essential. For children who experience difficulties with their sense of touch, hearing, or vision, occupational therapists (OTs) are often the best choice for diagnosis and therapy. Other experts would likely be able to detect sensory digestion problems as well. The following are included: ☐ Doctors who specialize in pediatrics and developmental-behavioral disorders. Psychologists, especially those specializing in neuropsychology.

Educational Assessors

Keeping an eye on your child's actions and reactions might help you see trends and triggers. However, knowing where to begin may be challenging.

Expert Assistance for Sensory Processing Disorders

When it comes to sensory processing disorders, there are

no treatments available. But there are a lot of professionals that can teach your child strategies to deal with sensory issues.

Kids with sensory difficulties are frequently seen in occupational therapy. They assist children in discovering ways to cope with sensory overload. Although Sensory Integration Therapy is a well-known treatment option, therapists often employ a strategy known as a sensory diet.

It is evident that that strategy is customized. Children can benefit from it by learning to relax and gain control over their emotions and actions. Because of this, they are better suited to learning and interacting with others.

Some examples of what might be part of a sensory diet are:

- Jacks that jump

- Jogging on a therapy ball

- Doing push-ups

- Leaping up and down slides

Heavy lifting, pushing or pulling against one's body, is a common theme among these pursuits.

Therapists that work with children often help those who struggle with sensory processing. Kids can get a lot of support talking through the feelings of anger and frustration brought on by their circumstances when they use Cognitive Behavioral Therapy.

Your child may be eligible for a 504 plan to help them with school-related adjustments. (Adjustments for sensory processing may also be part of your child's Individualized Education Program (IEP) if they have one for another concern.) The teacher may also provide your child with informal encouragement.

Some examples of classroom adjustments that can tremendously benefit students with sensory processing disorders are:

- Giving your child permission to use a fidget device.

- Offering a quiet area or earplugs for those who are

sensitive to noise.

- You can prepare your child for a significant change in routine by communicating this early on.

- Putting your child on a seat near open doors, windows, or whirling lights.

- Giving your child the option to self-regulate by considering exercise breaks.

Find further accommodations for challenges related to sensory digestion. Keep an eye on the steps to submit a 504 request for your child. Also, find out what to say to your child's teacher when they bring up sensory difficulties.

Some Strategies to Help Your Child Who Has Sensory Processing Disorder

The unexpected behaviors, especially sensory difficulties, could make life difficult for the family as a whole. However, by understanding their causes, one can discover ways to significantly alleviate their symptoms.

In and out of the house, you have a lot of options for tactics:

- Get strategies for avoiding trip meltdowns and find out how to make a sensory travel bundle.

- Investigate indoor pursuits that are gentler on the senses.

- Figure out what to do if your child refuses to wear winter clothes.

- For children who experience sensory difficulties, you can download a six-week vacation schedule.

Find out how to help your grade-schooler with their schoolwork.

Learn the basics of building self-advocacy in young children and how to guide students in elementary, middle, and high school as they figure it out for themselves. Find out simple ways to become your child's school advocate.

Chapter 3

Helpful Hints for Parents of Children with SPD

The disorder your child has in no way indicates anything about you as a parent. When we stop trying to figure out "why" or "how" things happened and just look at them as they are, we can find a much more natural and open perspective. The truth is that regular people, such as the parents of your children or friends of your family, will doubt your plan. While they may have a heart for helping, they lack the background and knowledge to effectively work with children who have sensory processing disorders. Stay the course! You and your family are the only ones who truly know what's best for your sensory child.

Put your wrath and guilt aside. Your ability to advocate for your sensory child will be severely impaired if you allow yourself to be consumed by feelings of blame, guilt, or wrath.

Appreciate the info that's already out there. As a parent of a sensory child, you should make it a routine to sit down and write down a few of the wonderful things you see and experience.

It could seem counterproductive to parent a child who is highly sensitive at first. It takes considerably more careful planning and thinking to father or mother a sensory child's day-to-day activities, which is why it might work while parenting most common kids normally doesn't. You can adapt your programs to deal with the day-to-day challenges that may arise if you can keep an eye on that one thought.

Embrace and appreciate your child's abilities. You should be well-versed in the benefits that your sensitive child enjoys. Make a list of all the wonderful things about your child. Not only are sensory kids unique, but they also happen to be some of the world's most accomplished adults. You should be prepared to encounter many people who fail to recognize or value their contributions.

Caring for a child with sensory processing disorder is

more like a marathon than a competition. Having a sensory child adds a lot of unexpected turns to the already exciting journey of parenthood. Keep the big picture in mind and make plans to achieve your long-term objectives.

Temporary sensory solutions do not exist. Your developing and ever-changing sensory child will require adjustments on a regular basis. Every child grows and evolves, but those with sensory processing disorders may find that these changes are particularly pronounced. You can discover solutions to the ever-changing challenges you may encounter with your sensitive youngster when you know how to use structure, routines, and visual aids.

When you mess up, brace yourself. As a result, you may learn more about how to help your sensitive child cope with challenging situations. Learn from the "incorrect" experiences.

Love and understanding ultimately lead the way. It is important for our sensory kids to know that they are loved and understood. Great youngsters who aren't quite sure how to navigate life on their own. They require and seek out daily opportunities to be in familiar surroundings, as this helps shape their perspective on the world. Doing this at home is within your capabilities.

So be it. Teaching sensory children how to use the equipment is one of the best long-term gifts we can give them. Starting to educate your sensitive child could pave the way for a lifetime of practice, the opportunity to learn from mistakes, and many forms of genuine success. A high school graduate who feels overwhelmed might pause and ask, "What's my purpose to take care of this or understand this done?" because this is essentially going to be their lifestyle. Independence (and good parenting) are actually characterized by this.

The Six Stages of Raising a Child with SPD

Refusing

Thinking about how his older sister never had "tantrums" that lasted several hours, I thought to myself, "Huh, This is actually the terrible twos," when he was two years old. I dubbed it "denial," and while there may have been some slight denial towards the end, I was still completely confused about how this behavior benefited him. My word is law.

Lack of Confidence in Oneself

All eyes were on me when I was three years old. Every day, the whole extended family went grocery shopping with us, and I took it upon myself to internalize his tantrums over my shortcomings, just like a parent would. His actions were a direct result of my mistakes, whether he was my sister, mother, or husband. The reality

Fury

Over the course of three or four years, I saw that my own anger against my child was rising. I had no idea how to appropriately react to him, and I had no idea why he acted in such a radical manner. Considering the widespread knowledge of the cognitive damage that might result from rage, I don't recall many worries throughout this round. I was overwhelmed by feelings of shame, resentment, and helplessness.

Understanding

I began to gather a mountain of information from the blogosphere, therapies, books, friends, and internet forums all at once. At this point, I focused on expanding my knowledge and building a network of people who understood the difficulties I was facing as a parent. For my second pocket, I required information and methods of contact.

Appreciating

I received an unexpected approval about five years ago. At this point, you've reached the "it really is just what it is usually" phase. Either I can make the most of the opportunities life has given me, or I may let myself be miserable, unfulfilled, and isolated from my husband, children, extended family, and friends. Accordingly, we would welcome his traits as gifts. Every day, he deals with challenging difficulties; yet, what truly makes his behavior distinctive and remarkable are the characteristics that push him towards it. He possesses exceptional professional functioning skills, is extremely organized, is very detail-oriented, and is fiercely loyal. His ability to understand people's emotions is evident. An adult with these traits is more likely to make deliberate choices, stand firm in his beliefs, and fight for what he believes in.

Achieving Success

You might find this step enjoyable. I had a new sense of assurance as a parent after completing the last stage and solving the situation. My current objective is to educate him on the reality that the very traits that make his life difficult also make it rich with opportunity and fulfillment. There is little hope for him to always be a happy, well-adjusted adult without acceptance of the qualities and appreciation of the attributes. Over and over, I will discover ways to accept his severe traits.

C h a p t e r   4

Children Deal with 15 Different Types of Sensory Processing Disorders

1.Extremely Sensitive

Extreme heightened sensitivity to stimuli is a hallmark of sensory over-responsive condition in children. In contrast to the average individual, they may be more prone to becoming overly sensitive whenever their senses are aroused. A child with this type of sensory impairment may experience aversions to touch, loud noises, bright lights, or strong flavors.

A state of "sensory defensiveness" could develop in these kids if they're overstimulated in any way. Nervousness, heart palpitations, sweating, trembling, and adrenaline rushes are common symptoms of sensory defensiveness, which is often a "battle or air travel" reaction.

Reducing or eliminating exposure to potentially overwhelming levels of stimulation is the gold standard treatment for children with sensory over-responsive condition.

Because of the lower class sizes, quieter classrooms, and lack of distractions caused by large numbers of students, he may thrive at an exclusive or charter school. Children with this illness can learn to manage circumstances that overwhelm their senses via therapy and go on to lead fully healthy lives.

2. Lack of Sensory Reactivity

Sensory under-responsive disorder (SUD) children may experience the polar opposite of sensory over-responsive disorder (SOD) children. They seem to have emerged as quiet and submissive, or they show up all withdrawn and self-absorbed.

Because there are more people around, children with this disease don't perceive sensory inputs as strongly. This is why a child with sensory under-responsive ness could not feel the seasons or discomfort as much as other children their age. Because she lacks the normal tactile sensitivity, she sustains cuts, scratches, bumps, and bruises without ever knowing it or feeling the agony.

Clumsiness, frequent falling, and bumping into objects are all symptoms that children with sensory under-responsive condition may exhibit. This is because, due to their impaired body awareness, these kids have a hard time perceiving their environment.

3. Appetite Snatching

Kids who suffer from sensory seeking disorder are constantly on the lookout for new and exciting experiences. A child suffering from sensory seeking disorder may have trouble understanding the importance of personal space and may have an overwhelming need for physical contact with others at all times. His want to live was always strong, and he could sense everything around him, as well as dash into surfaces and leap around.

In the case of a sensory problem, the most aggravating aspect is certainly the fact that stimulus does not relax the child but rather makes him seek it more. Oftentimes, doctors would diagnose ADD or ADHD in children who exhibit sensory seeking disorder signs.

The symptoms of Sensory Craving Disorder might

manifest in a child's compulsive need to constantly explore, touch, run, bump, and crash. Though some psychologists are hesitant to diagnose a child with sensory craving disorder apart from attention deficit hyperactivity disorder (ADHD) or attention deficit disorder (ADD), others believe that a child can be told they have sensory craving disorder even if neither of those conditions is present. More study and observation is needed to clarify if a child can be diagnosed with Sensory Craving Disorder in the absence of an ADD or ADHD evaluation, or if sensory craving disorder is a symptom associated with these illnesses. The medical profession is divided on the matter.

4. Poor Posture

Because they lack control over their eye and inner movements, children with postural disorder may appear sluggish, but they may actually have trouble standing up straight and sitting up straight. Symptoms of postural dysfunction can vary and include a generalized slouching and occasional leaning on objects or people, an unwillingness to participate in physical activities, weak muscles, decreased quantities of energy, and overall weariness.

Because he or she avoids situations where they have to move about, a child with this illness runs the risk of being socially isolated. For fear of falling, appearing foolish, or being unable to continue, children with this disease frequently withdraw from video games or activities. Since they have a hard time sitting up straight in class, they grow tired and have trouble focusing, which could lead them to fall behind in college.

There is a treatment for postural problem. Motivating children with this sensory condition to be active is important. They get over their lack of coordination and balance once some time has passed and are able to develop their main muscles. Children with postural disorders can benefit from therapy in order to receive the support they require for a successful outcome.

5. Spelling problems

It is difficult for children with dyspraxia to properly interpret sensory data. This means that a child with dyspraxia may have problems with goal-setting, visual planning, and learning new motor skills. A child who has difficulty with speech may also be clumsy and prone to accidents. It's likely that she may struggle to complete tasks that need exceptional motor abilities. Some sports, particularly those involving throwing or catching a ball, may be challenging for her, and she may also damage playthings. She might try to hide her problem by avoiding things she knows will be difficult for her, like a sore thumb. Dream play is another possible activity for her to engage in, since it is a place where she feels free to learn and develop without ever having to face the consequences of her choices.

Children with dyspraxia may benefit greatly from therapy, as mentioned before. Children with dyspraxia may have to put in more effort to succeed at things that other kids take for granted. However, just as with any other talent, the more time and effort put into perfecting a skill, the easier it will be for them to use.

6. Auditory

Central auditory processing disorder (APD) is a developmental disorder in which a child has trouble understanding what sounds they hear. When there are undoubtedly a lot of things going on, he may struggle to discern subtle changes in voice modulation or individual sounds. Although they may have no problems hearing or completing tasks when alone in a quiet room, children with this disease may struggle to understand and follow directions when there is a lot going on around them.

Helping children diagnosed with this disease is of the utmost importance. Young people who suffer from auditory processing disorders can, with time and treatment, develop normal attention and processing skills.

Untreated sensory processing disorder can cause a child to lag behind in school in a variety of subjects, including but not limited to: language, reading, writing, vocabulary, and conversation.

Up to five percent of kids may have auditory processing disorder. Auditory processing disorder might develop in a child if he or she has trouble following directions, becomes quickly distracted by loud or unexpected sounds, or becomes irritated in environments with a lot of background noise.

7. Visual

It can be difficult for a child with visual control disorder to make sense of information that is processed by the eyes. She has a tendency to mix up letters b and d, get distracted easily, spill food or drinks, and accidentally bump against people or objects. She might also have trouble processing varied distances or determining the proximity or distance of an object to her.

One type of learning disability is dyslexia, while another is visual processing disorder. Again, opinions vary as to whether the two diseases will be identical or wholly separate.

For a student with Visual Control Disorder to succeed in college, therapy may play a crucial role.

Early diagnosis of the condition and access to child care while connections are being established are the key features. The earlier a child's condition is identified, the better their chances of successfully overcoming it.

8. Sensitivity to Touch Defense

A child who is tactilely defensive will be far more sensitive to physical touch than the average person. Simple things that many of us don't even think about could end up bothering him. Things that can irritate a child with tactile defensiveness include, but are not limited to, rough textures, things that are perceived as "messy," vibrating objects, physical contact (such as hugs and kisses), clothing tags, bedsheets, dirt or grime, grass or mud on bare feet, wind, blowing on exposed skin, and shoes.

An uninterested child may use the tips of his fingers to explore different textures, such as sand, food, play-doh, glitter, or color. It is possible that tactile defensiveness is affecting the majority of children in this situation. When he has to put on his shoes and socks, he may scream or cry.

It is possible to control and eventually conquer this

illness with therapy. Recognizing a child's difficulties with tactile defensiveness is generally the first step. There are a plethora of options for treating and combating the illness once this is determined.

9. The vestibular system

Among the five senses that humans are aware of, the vestibular system is among the most important. The vestibular system, which originates in the inner ear's fluid, helps in stability, coordination, and good vision.

Because of difficulties with hypo or hyper vestibular control, a child with vestibular processing dysfunction may appear clumsy, lethargic, hyperactive, or impulsive. Any activity that requires the feet to be active, such swinging, slipping, monkey bars, riding a bike, or climbing, may be appealing to a child with the hyperactive type of this illness. A child coping with hypo shape may hate, avoid, or dread these things regardless of the circumstances.

Some people with vestibular processing impairment feel lightheaded very quickly, whereas others don't feel lightheaded at all after very vigorous spinning. These people may also favor motionless activities or enjoy the sensation of whirling, rocking, or tilting. Treatment is highly effective once a child has received a diagnosis of this disease.

10. The ability to detect movements

Having proprioception means you can feel your own body's position in space. Indeed, it is the determinant of the appropria te amount of force to apply while opening a door or lifting a laundry basket. Children who suffer from Proprioceptive Digestive Disorder may struggle to maintain their body's natural alignment, control their gait, and determine the appropriate amount of force to apply in different contexts.

Some symptoms that may indicate that a child is struggling with this disorder include: leg kicking or jumping while sitting and heavy foot stomping while walking; enjoying the sensation of pressure when wrapped in a warm blanket or lying underneath a heavy object; pushing too hard when coloring or writing;

engaging in too rough of play with peers; and occasionally dropping or spilling objects.

Treatment can help a child with this disease overcome some of the symptoms. Perhaps the best treatment for a child with this issue would be to send him or her to a playground where they can work on their spatial awareness.

The fact that parents are happy to have their children help out around the house with things like washing clothes or mowing the lawn—tasks that require lifting, dragging, or pushing—is another excellent therapy.

11. Exempt from

A child's ability to taste is affected by Gustatory Processing Disorder. This condition manifests itself in a child's heightened sensitivity to taste or inability to control what she puts in her mouth.

Some of the symptoms that may indicate that a child has this illness include an extreme aversion to eating certain foods, a strong gag reflex, excessive drooling, and an incessant need to chew on objects (such as pens, toys, or t-shirt sleeves). A child with this illness could have strong feelings about teeth brushing, the taste of toothpaste, or even the dentist, or she could have strong feelings about all three. Asking her to try new foods, particularly those with strong flavors or textures, makes her anxious.

For children with gustatory processing dysfunction, the best things to do include giving them crunchy or chewy snacks throughout the day, toys that appear like they use their jaws, such kazoos or bubbles, and hard candies with strong sweet or sour flavors.

12. A sense of smell

Problems with smell-related tasks are common among children n with olfactory control dysfunction. Some or all of the following symptoms may be displayed by a child with this disorder: an interest in smelling scented things (such as soap, gas, or lotions), an aversion to smells (which most people can't detect), a reluctance to try new foods because of their smell, an obsession with how someone else smells when deciding whether they like them, and an extreme dislike of strong fragrances (such as those found in perfumes, colognes, or lotions).

Many options exist for assisting a child with this illness. Help kids pick up on the fact that fragrances are essential to their environment. Recognize new smells daily and talk about their origins and whether or not a child enjoys them. Once this condition is recognized, a child who feels his complaints about smells are being acknowledged may benefit greatly from the knowledge that others understand his struggles. As previously said, the first line of defense against sensory problems is early detection and treatment.

Problems with interoceptive processing can make it hard for a child to control their bodily functions, including their ability to sleep, urinate, eat, consume, and even breathe properly during yoga. She might despise the sense of hunger and eat frequently to relieve it, or she might use frequent restroom breaks to stave off the urge to go to the bathroom. She may also like the feelings of hunger and the desire to control her portion sizes, which can lead her to overeat and undereat at inappropriate times and to ignore the need to use the restroom when she really needs to. Malnutrition or bladder contamination may follow these actions.

When it comes to slumber, the same is true. Children suffering from this condition may either sleep excessively or very little. They might attempt to hold their breath because the sensation is uncomfortable, or they might think about taking deep breaths because they enjoy the sensation of air moving through their lungs.

It is difficult to manage with this condition in any of its manifestations. Each of these tasks is essential for daily living, and parents may find themselves becoming increasingly frustrated with a child who has difficulty with any of them. Keep calm and ask for assistance. This condition is also quite curable. With the right help, any kid can do it.

14. A Combination of Both

Each case of sensory impairment is unique. Despite this, the issue is becoming more understood and diagnosable, and there are many children with sensory impairments who are thriving despite the challenges they face.

Difficulty levels range from moderate to severe, and symptoms can be quite different from one disorder to the next. A child may experience difficulties with up to eight distinct sensory issues simultaneously, and they may also experience difficulties with different subtypes within each of the eight main categories.

Psychologists and occupational therapists who work with children who have sensory processing disorders are experts at making individualized diagnoses based on patterns seen in their patients. Just as no two children are ever the same, no two cases of children with sensory impairments are ever the same. When given a specific medication, children have very little to fear.

15. Condition Varying in Severity

Autism is more common in boys than girls. While 1 in 142 children have autism spectrum disorder, just 1 in 189 females have.

A wide range of symptoms, from mild to severe, make up autism spectrum disorder. Many autistic youngsters also struggle with sensory processing issues. While some medical professionals and psychologists mistakenly assume that a child with a sensory issue also has autism, others maintain that the two conditions are distinct.

No matter what, it's important to love, support, and be patient with any youngster who is trying to seem reasonable in the face of overwhelming external pressures. For kids, this relatively recent cluster of illnesses could spell disaster. Thankfully, studies have been carried out, therapies are being created, and our understanding of sensory issues and how to manage them continues to grow daily.

Seek assistance if you become aware that a child you know is dealing with a sensory disorder. A battling child's chances of living a long, healthy life improve in proportion to the speed with which therapy is initiated.

Strategies to Help Students with SPDs Stay Engaged in Class

Symptoms of sensory processing disorder can include an inability to properly interpret information from many senses, including touch, hearing, and smell. Given the potential for both hypersensitivity and hyposensitivity, it may be difficult for parents and teachers to exert control.

Based on my experience in pediatrics, which spans over a decade, I can attest to the fact that classroom performance is dramatically improved when teachers possess a deeper comprehension of the unique needs of these students. So, before you can figure out how to help your scholar, you need to know which category they fit under.

An intolerance

A child like this one will go to great lengths to avoid any kind of sensory input. From the sound of the hand dryers in the restroom comes the cries of a little child who seems to be in agony. Some of the statements they make are:

- "Take it from me!It's possible that kids have a very sensitive sense of smell, especially when it comes to clothing details like seams or brands. They may be so attached to a certain T-shirt that they won't let anything change their mind about it, or they may insist on wearing garments backwards so they can avoid the sensation of sure stitching. When you have to worry about your nails or hair, grooming can become even more of a chore.

- "It's painful!" "One thing every day seems or looks "damaged" to children with sensitivities. It could be the noise from the vacuum cleaner or the light from the table lamp.

- I hate it! Children may also be put off by unpleasant odors. A specific eating regimen may be necessary if foods that do not upset some people trigger gag reflexes in these.

- Please, don't touch me. Children that are hypersensitive should not be handled or hugged because it could make them feel uncomfortable. Additionally, they may be put off by the sound of group play and warily withdraw from a business. Children with SPD may find the activity levels of group play to be too high.

Hyposensitivity symptoms

Among them are the children who crave constant stimulation and are always looking for new adventures. The fact that he didn't feel or respond to cutting himself is what will amaze you when this child returns from your playground. Common indicators include:

- "Oh no!" When providing sensory feedback, hyposensitive children frequently act irritated, bite, or scratch themselves.

- "Oops!"Hyposensitive children have trouble gauging distance and authority, which manifests as awkwardness or unfamiliarity when interacting with other people in their private spaces. This means they have problems sitting still, slam doors more strongly than necessary, and frequently collide with other individuals. To keep comfortable examples of stimulation, they may even need movement and activities.

- "Right away, without delay!This form of SPD makes children more likely to eat too quickly, which increases their risk of choking. Furthermore, moving from one task to another is a challenge.

Keep in mind that many of the symptoms may also point to other conditions. For instance, ADD/ADHD may explain why autistic children frequently prefer to play alone, and the associated avoidance of social interaction may be a symptom of autism itself. That's a difficulty for diagnosis, and with teacher guidance, we can isolate the underlying structure of the behaviors to consult with other specialists.

Making a Difference in the Lives of Children with Sensory Processing Disorder via Construction

The inability of the brain to properly interpret incoming channels of information is characteristic of Sensory Processing Disorder, formerly known as Sensory

Integration Dysfunction. Individuals affected by this illness, whether they are children or adults, may have a significantly harder time meeting their basic needs due to their heightened or diminished sensitivity to sensory inputs.

Unfortunately, there is currently no accepted diagnosis for SPD, and so, it may be difficult to seek treatment for the disorder. But Dr. Leah Light of the Brainchild Institute in Hollywood, Florida, is adamant that they are available. If you know a parent whose child pulls their clothes off because it's too itchy, covers their ears because the noises are too crazy, or gags when a toothbrush is placed in their mouth, you might want to ask them about Sensory Digestive Disorder. Perhaps you'll get an enthusiastic "yes!" "She makes it clear that she is aware.

Children who experience typical reactions to their sensory settings may perceive the world as a frightening place. Perhaps parents too feel apprehensive about it. Whenever a child with SPD has consistent difficulties with everyday tasks and meltdowns, it becomes increasingly difficult to choose where to begin. Regardless, you must be able to assist your child. Breathe deeply and take charge.

If you want to help your child overcome their difficulties, you need to know their likes, dislikes, and what sets them off.

Do You Think Your Child Is More of a Sensory Seeker or Avoider?

Light argues that children whose sensory systems are more sensitive to stimuli have a higher threshold for perceiving information, distinguishing them from children whose sensory systems are less sensitive. Consequently, people are seeking further information in order to understand the message they wish to receive. Conversely, those who choose to avoid sensory experiences do so because they have lower sensory thresholds, which means that even a small quantity of transmission might elicit a strong response. Arousal is too much for them, therefore they try to avoid it. Hyperactive behaviors can be exhibited by both sensory seekers and sensory avoiders, but for distinct causes, as Light elucidates. "The one on the left is trying to get more insight and work toward the stimulus, while the one on the right is trying to get less insight and work through the stimulus."

According to Light, children who are sensory avoiders—those who are easily startled by certain sounds, lights, or smells—may find comfort in activities that put a lot of pressure on their skin, challenge their muscles, or reveal their bones. On the flip side, children who seek out sensory experiences tend to be hyperactive. In order to explore as many options as possible for stepping, falling, crashing, kicking, drawing, pushing, suspending, lifting, etc., they frequently react positively to extremely intense forms of sensory stimulation.

Keep in mind that your child is unique, not only from other children but also from many other children with SPD. Some children may be very emotionally reactive, some may seek out sensory experiences, and yet others may exhibit a combination of the two. They'll appreciate some things and despise others; the goal is to gain wisdom via trial and error. Where they travel, what they do, who they're with, etc., can all affect your child's patterns.

At the end of the day, a game of elimination might help you figure out what makes your child feel secure and happy, and then you can provide them chances to put those ideas into practice. For example, you may need to take a few minutes each day to bounce around on a mini-trampoline or use noise-cancelling headphones while you study. When you have a general idea of your child's demands, you can adjust your daily activities and household routines to meet those needs.

Ways to Make Your Home More Engaging for Those Who Seek Meaning via Sight and Touch

• *Try using a weighted vest, blanket, or toy.*

Moving furniture, vacuuming, carrying the laundry basket, and digging in the garden are all examples of indoor and outdoor tasks that your child may help you with.

Play the "sandwich game" with your child, where they lie between two cushions and you ask them, "Harder or softer?" at varying pressures to see which one they prefer.with each press.

- To enhance flavor, provide meals that are chewy, sour, or spicy.

- All the way up your child's limbs, provide "embracing squeezes," which are really just deep pressure squeezes.

- Toys made of rubber, such as racquetballs, are great for children.

- Put your child in garments that fit snugly and have elastic waistbands.

Toy towel tug-of-war is a lot of fun.

- Take your child to the park and let him play on the hills or climb trees.

- Give your child a head massage or a weighted cap before a trip to the dentist or hairdresser if they have trouble calming down during those appointments. Put your child's books in a backpack and let them wear it while you run errands.

Methods for Using Your Sensory Avoider to Bring Sensory Insight into Your Regular Routine

- Let your child run their hands through some dry mud or grain; this will encourage them to explore and learn. Instruct them to uncover hidden riches by covering a large area with mud or grain.

Testing with splashing, pouring, and regular water is possible with these containers.

- As the clock ticks down to victory, put on some relaxing music and encourage your child to get moving.

- Involve your child in the process of making the ingredient, dough, or meat tenderizer. They can also help you bring in the necessary pots, pans, and ingredients.

- While your child is in the shower, use a washcloth or shower brush to gently scrub their skin. Apply multiple soaps and lotions. Next, make a wall structure out of shaving cream or shower foam. Finally, sprinkle powder on your child's body and massage it into their skin.

- Hold and cuddle your child frequently. Softly stroke their hair, face, and ears with a variety of textures, such as cotton balls, vibrating massagers, and feathers.

- Light suggests that in a calm, undisturbed environment, sensory avoiders should be exposed to just one type of stimulus at a time.

If you want to help make adjustments to their normal routine or conduct unexpected duties, be sure to let them know in the mandated time. Many kids with SPD need predictability.

According to the Celebrity Institute for Sensory Control

Disorder, it is crucial that you recognize the symptoms of your child's current overstimulation. Unexpected yawning, hiccups, burping, changes in the skin, excessive overactivity, and dangerous or foolish behavior in excess are all examples of such things. Do what helps to calm your child down—for example, putting them in a blanket, holding them and rocking them gently, or giving them a warm shower—if you see these specific things. Stop the knowledge immediately.

Here are six ways you may support your child who has a sensory processing disorder.

The brain and the senses are at the center of Sensory Processing Disorder, which is also known as Sensory Control Disorder. This mental state is characterized by difficulty in controlling and making sense of one's own ideas.

In common parlance, SPD is often understood as a disorder in which the brain has problems processing and making sense of sensory input, according to a WebMD explanation.

How can you help your child cope with each disorder?

There are four distinct kinds of SPDs, or sensory processing disorders:

- Visible—associated with the faculty of seeing

- Auditory — associated with hearing

- Odor - associated with taste and smell (nose, throat)

- Tactile — connected to the flesh (fingertips)

Let's take a look at each type and see how you can assist your child in dealing with them.

Persistent Visual Impairment

Inputs associated with vision are problematic for children suffering from Visual Sensory Control Disorder. Some approaches to help children who are struggling with these issues are as follows:

Children that have visual sensory processing disorder often have trouble maintaining eye contact, therefore it's important to be gentle while dealing with them. As a general rule, when they're speaking to you, you shouldn't make them look at you. If you insist that they know you for sure, they can lose concentration. Explain that it's alright to never look at you, break the issue down into its component parts, and give them a chance to process what they're hearing instead. Show people where to look if you have something on show.

Shiny lights could be disturbing, therefore anything having to do with lighting should be considered. Be careful to adjust the lighting and illumination settings appropriately. To soothe the eyes, try a variety of low-light options that aren't too gloomy. For kids who find the sun too much to bear, a good pair of sunglasses can be just what they need. Even while they're in school, they should ask their professor to put their desk in a special, shaded spot.

- Minimize visual distractions: a plethora of colors could be harsh on the eyes and make it difficult to concentrate. To ensure a restful night's sleep, decorate their room with soft hues and keep everything neat and tidy.

Problems with Hearing and Balance

Some children have trouble hearing because they have a Sound Sensory Control Disorder that is associated with loud noises. Sounds, such as those produced by a drilling machine or an airplane, can be difficult for them to handle, but this helps.

Here are a few ways to assist kids who are facing these kinds of challenges:

- Before you take your child out, make sure they are aware of what sounds they can encounter and how to behave appropriately in certain situations. Get them ready ahead of time so that no amount of noise will scare them; even a high-quality car horn could annoy them.

- Keep earplugs, noise-cancelling headphones, etc., on hand at all times; this will help muffle potentially dangerous sounds. To discover the ideal ear protection for your child, you may need to try out a few different types.

- Novel experiences: Taking your child outside exposes them to a wide variety of sounds, none of which are likely to be appealing to them. Calling ahead to find out when the store has a less crowd could be helpful if you want to take your child to a supermarket or electronics showroom. Your child is welcome to accompany you on certain days going forward.

Problems with Smell and Taste Sensitivity

Personal scent preferences and difficulties with olfactory and flavor processing may manifest in children with sensory processing disorders. Some people may have sensitivities to certain foods or scents, such as some plants or dairy.

Some ways to assist kids with these kinds of problems are listed below:

- Be vigilant about food allergies: your child may be experiencing unique flavors that change from one season to the next. The things they consume have a major impact on their daily routine. Each move has an immediate impact on their eating, so it's smart to keep an eye on that.

- Make sense of the connection between fragrance and flavor: It's hard to think of a situation where aroma and flavor aren't related. Our sense of smell can deduce the chemical from the flavor, and our taste receptors can tell us what kind it is. This is the main reason why youngsters who are sensitive to flavors rely so much on fragrance.

- A brief flavor profile: Children who have food allergies should not have the same meal every day. Introducing things to people with different tastes and interests is crucial. Set the dish out in front of them and ease their transition to the original recipe by revealing components; this will allow them to pick out the ones they enjoy best.

A Disorder of the Tactile Nerve

True issue-related Sensory Control Disorders manifest as

a persistent aversion to physical touch in children. As an added complication, these are easily irritated and overpowered by physical touch, and they are sensitive to specific materials.

Some ways to assist kids with these kinds of problems are listed below:

- *Take them shopping:* Let them choose the cloth that they like most. Also, make sure to let them use the sheets they like. Everything they come into contact with should be suitable and gentler on their skin.

- *Physical touch:* When it comes to youngsters who are tactilely sensitive, nothing delights them more than when someone brushes their hair or presses against them. Get your kid(s) ready before you decide to give them a haircut or take care of their grooming needs.

If your child has a tactile sensitivity, it may be difficult, if not impossible, to give them a firm embrace, therefore it's important to find alternative ways to express your love. That doesn't imply you can't express your affection in other ways. All it takes is a little conversation, a gentle touch of your hand (with their permission), and the cloth they want to feel.

Chapter 5

What You Should Know Before Dating Someone Who Has Sensory Processing Disorder

You have this direct influence over your emotions and the precise way you connect with people; picture a world devoid of sounds, images, and touches. Envision yourself waking up two years from now, getting a pair of scissors, and taking the tags off every article of clothing you've owned. Picture yourself protecting your ear each time a fire engine passes by. How would you like to handle the sensation of clothes tags constantly scratching at your flesh, making it itch like hell or even feel like it's burning? Envision yourself dating someone with Sensory Control Disorder (SPD), a condition characterized by intense experiences with several senses. If you're involved with such a unique and wonderful individual, I have some dating tips for you.

1. Change your frame of thought

Know that your companion is an individual, just like yourself, and that you are distinct from everyone else on Earth. What should one do ultimately? You should keep in mind that you have the option to change your approach, visit locations over the day, or even alter the way you touch your partner. These differences may be hard for some people to understand, but for others, they provide a once-in-a-lifetime chance to connect with someone special.

2. Sense of Spidey!

People really do possess eight senses. They might be:

- Olfactory system (smell)

- Visual system (view)

- Tactile System (touch)

- Gustatory System (taste)

- Auditory System (audio)

- Proprioceptive system (body consciousness)

- The vestibular system (balance)

- Interceptive System (state of organs).

Even though there are eight senses in total, it's important to keep in mind that every adult with SPD experiences a different variety of sensations. Consequently, their sensitivity could be off in one or more senses. Someone with a high threshold for sound may enjoy going to a concert, whereas someone with a lower threshold may need to set an interval limit so they don't get confused. Because the stimulus is so large and powerful, some people want to avoid this particular event. Perhaps a pact is the best way to involve your partner in your plans. So that kids aren't too distracted by all the noise from the machines and other people talking, you could ask the gym manager if there is a less busy time of day. (Your friend can, in fact, feel multiple stimuli at once and tyre out quickly!) To get a feel for each other's similarities, differences, and thresholds, I recommend having a pre-date conversation and taking note of your partner's senses. Indulging in this romantic interaction enables both individuals to be informed about upcoming activities and creates additional opportunities for shared, unforgettable encounters.

3. Accept and Embrace Your Uncomfortable

A person learns more from a single mistake than from a string of advantages, at least in my experience. For example, in order for you to comprehend the preferred method of care for someone with SPD, it is likely that both of you will need to adjust. Please tell me what this means. For your partner, touch—particularly constant, localized caressing—may seem like a scorching sensation. Let me be clear: it doesn't mean you or your partner end up completely devastated. We still don't know how to feel about what is right and what is tolerable. Both sides have a chance to connect on a magical level and openly express their current emotions in the previously mentioned situation. On top of that, it makes it possible to build relationships. She may express, "I really like what you are really doing, nonetheless it could experience better if you'd vary how you handled me and the positioning, i.e., light, hard, kneading, etc. -- on my arm." Totally, act erratically. Just a kind reminder that everyone is different and that these kinds of things might happen; nonetheless, staying in constant and quick contact might help you and your spouse stay connected and on the same page.

4. As in, via the abdominal cavity

Your pet may benefit from a special feeding regimen that helps them maintain a healthy internal environment. Instead of sabotaging it by insisting on going to restaurants that the typical person cannot afford, at least be helpful. I encourage you to engage with the new menu items and try something different. You may show your partner how much you care by trying a new, tasty cuisine, and you can improve your health by eating more whole, natural foods.

5. Have a long-term view

Because your partner's experiences tend to change, it's important to check in with them on a regular basis to assess their level. Realize that, depending on their findings, previously agreed-upon programs may have to be delayed or canceled. Keep in mind that it's quite normal if your pet becomes too excited. When this happens, your skill is to give them space to regulate themselves, because everyone has a unique method of doing so. "Experience is only the name we give our errors," Oscar Wilde once published. Be mindful of this. Amass knowledge. As you bask in the company of wonderful, wonderful people right now.

Create Your Own Sensory Bottle

Is your child hyperactive, has trouble regulating their emotions, or has trouble focusing? Even if you try to calm her down, she can still have problems if that's the case. A sensory container could be useful if your child has trouble focusing on one thing due to too many stimuli. Kids will learn to control their impulses with the help of this musical instrument. The term "neural tube" may describe it. The fact that a sensory bottle is a calm, focused object is crucial for children. Another option would be for her to shake her head in order to gain a solid proprioceptive understanding. In addition, we will experiment with different sensory containers to captivate her interest.

The specific materials needed to create your handmade sensory container may vary with the bottle you pick, but here are the absolute minimum:

The following materials are needed:

- Warm water

- Glitter • Food coloring

- A funnel

- Superglue (or a hot glue gun)

- A clean, empty, typical water bottle made of plastic (with the label removed)

Simplified corn syrup

Crafting a Glitter-Inspired Themed Sensory Basket

- You can whip up this dazzling sensory bottle in no time. As your child shakes it or holds it in her hands, she will experience visual calm. Plus, it may be tailored to your child's interests, making it that much more appealing. Use blue food color, blue glitter, and confetti shaped like seafood if your child likes the water.

- Start by squeezing some corn syrup into a clean water bottle. Use enough syrup to fill the jar one-third of the way. (Although the video up above uses corn syrup, you may try using essential oils.) Approximately three quarters of the way filled, add hot water. The next step is to add a few drops of food colorant and glitter. After adding the components to the water container, cover it and shake to combine.

- Fill the container as full as possible with drinking water once you're satisfied with the appearance. Reapply the lid and use hot glue or superglue to keep it in place.

Constructing a Vibrational Sensory Bottle

- Fill a clean water container up to three quarters of the way with water for drinking. Add a few drops of food coloring. When the food dye has dispersed in the water, add the infant gas or cooking gas to the remaining containers.

- Use superglue to fasten the cover. To get your child interested in seeing how oil and water separate, you can set the container on its base and let them shake it to simulate waves.

Turning Sand into a "Peekaboo" Sensory JarFor both visual and tactile cues, try using a "peekaboo" sensory bottle. Your child may also find it easier to focus.

Make this bottle out of colored play sand or rice that has been painted with food coloring (there are many of recipes online).

Fill a clean water jug halfway with mud or grain and place a funnel inside. Include little toys, such as alphabet beads, LEGO pieces, or mini-erasers.After that, fill up the remaining bottles with mud or rice, making sure to leave about an inch of space at the top. This will allow the material to bypass and become confused. Before you use superglue to seal the lid, give the container a good shake.

The container could be a great tool for your sensory-seeking child to use for a lot of tasks. As she spins it around, searching for particular people or things, the weight of it may be a comfort.

Acknowledgements

Behold the magnificent triumph of this extraordinary book, a testament to the divine intervention of God Almighty and the unwavering love and support of my cherished Family, devoted Fans, avid Readers, loyal Customers, and dear Friends. Their ceaseless encouragement has paved the way for this resounding success.

www.ingramcontent.com/pod-product-compliance
Lightning Source LLC
Chambersburg PA
CBHW031133020426
42333CB00012B/351